# Contents

Preface..................................................................2
Reception.............................................................5
Anamnesis..........................................................11
Massage..............................................................23
Manual therapy..................................................28
PNF.....................................................................38
Mulligan.............................................................44
Exercises............................................................47
Gait Training.....................................................54
Lymphatic drainage..........................................56
Electrotherapy...................................................60
Pelvic floor exercises........................................63
Breathing therapy.............................................67
Useful.................................................................70
Thanks................................................................72
Bibliography......................................................73

# Preface

**Who am I?**

My name is Caroline Braun and I created the Little Physio.
I studied translation and worked as a freelance translator.
I then decided to change my way of living and became a physiotherapist / physical therapist.
I've been working as a physical therapist for over 10 years in different hospitals as well as in private practices.

**Why did I create Little Physio?**

My experience has shown me the difficulties of treating patients who don't speak the same language.
It's difficult and even sometimes impossible to diagnose or treat the patient correctly.
The consequences for the patient are disastrous.

Many people think that the patient has to speak the language of the country he or she lives in.
Even if correct it's also not always possible.
Some people are not able to learn or have just arrived.
Others might be on vacation or are only here temporarily to work.

I am a physical therapist and my job is not to judge but to treat the patients.
And I have to treat them the best I can.

That's why I created "Little Physio".

**This translator enables the therapist to communicate and to treat foreign patients.**

Your therapy will become easier and better.

The book is divided into 14 chapters like "Reception", "Massage", "Manual therapy", "Exercises" and so on. This makes it easier and faster for you to find the sentences you need.

**In addition to the book**, you have the opportunity to get the **Little Physio App for mobile phones and tabs, iphone and ipad.**

The Apps are available on the Apple Appstore and on the Googleplaystore.

The **Little Physio Apps are the audio version of the books**.

It is as easy as clicking on the needed sentence and your cell phone or tab "speaks" it out in the foreign language.

You can see a demo on:

littlephysio.com

or on

youtube

I became a physical therapist to help others, no matter if they speak my language or not.

**Now, it is possible!**

# Reception

Accoglienza

**1. Hello**
Buon giorno

**2. My name is**
Mi chiamo

**3. Do you have a doctor's prescription?**
Ha una ricetta del dottore?

**4. Yes**
Si

**5. No**
No

**6. Do you have your insurance card?**
Ha il libretto assicurativo?

**7. Would you please bring the insurance card next time?**

Lo può portare la prossima volta?

**8. Would you please write down your phone number?**

Mi scrive il suo numero di telefono per favore?

**9. There is a mistake in the prescription. You have to go back to your doctor and have him issue a new one.**

Qui c´é un sbaglio sulla ricetta per piacere vada di nuovo dal dottore, a chiedergli una ricetta nuova.

**10. Do you have a report / X-ray / CT- images from your doctor?**

Ha un rapporto / Radiografia, TAC del dottore?

**11. Would you please bring the x-rays / the report with you next time?**

La prossima volta mi porti il rapporto, le radiografie?

**12. Here are your appointments**

Questi sono i suoi appuntamenti

**13. If these appointments can't work for you, please let me know.**

Se li appuntamenti non vanno bene per lei, melo dica.

**14. This one doesn't work?**

Qui non vá?

**15. Not on this day at all?**

Questo giorno non vá?

**16. Rather in the morning?**

Meglio di mattina?

**17. Rather in the afternoon?**

Meglio di pomeriggio?

**18. Monday**

Lunedì

**19. Tuesday**

Martedì

**20. Wednesday**
Mercoledì

**21. Thursday**
Giovedì

**22. Friday**
Venerdì

**23. Saturday**
Sabato

**24. Sunday**
Domenica

**25. I'm sorry, you are too early**
Mi dispiace, ma lei è in anticipo

**26. I'm sorry, you are too late**
Mi dispiace, ma lei è in ritardo

**27. This week won't work**

Questa settimana non vá

**28. Today doesn't work**

Oggi non vá

**29. Not before next week**

La prossima settimana

**30. Not before next month**

Il prossimo mese

**31. The therapist is on vacation**

Il terapista é in vacanze

**32. The therapist is ill**

Il terapista é malato

**33. Would you like to work with a different therapist?**

Vuole andare da un altro terapista?

**34. Yes**

Si


**35. No**

No


**36. Would you like to continue with the same therapist?**

Desidera lo stesso terapista?


**37. Would you rather wait until your therapist is back?**

Vuole aspettare finché arriva il terapista?


**38. Here is your bill.**

Qui é il suo conto


**39. Would you like to pay now?**

Vuole pagare adesso?


**40. Do you want to pay cash?**

Vuole pagare in contanti?

# Anamnesis

Anamnesi

**1. Please undress**
Si spogli per favore

**2. Can you please take off your top ?**
Può togliersi il disopra?

**3. Can you please take off your pants?**
Può togliersi il pantalone?

**4. Can you please take off your skirt?**
Può togliersi la gonna?

**5. Are you in pain?**
Ha dei dolori?

**6. Yes**
Si

**7. No**
No

**8. Show me where it hurts**
Mi faccia vedere dove ha dolori

**9. Where does it hurt?**
Dove ha dolori?

**10. Is the pain radiating into your arm?**
Vanno per il braccio?

**11. Is the pain radiating into your leg?**
Vanno nella gamba?

**12. Where does the pain radiate into?**
Fino dove arrivanno i dolori?

**13. Show me**
Mi faccia vedere

**14. Do you feel numbness?**
Sente la mancanza di sensibilità?

**15. Where?**
Dove?

**16. Do you have paralytic symptoms?**
Ha dei sindromi di paralizzo?

**17. Do you feel formication?**
Ha dei formicolii?

**18. Where?**
Dove?

**19. When did it start?**
Da quando?

**20. For days**
Da giorni

**21. For weeks**
Da settimane

**22. For months**
Da mesi

**23. For years**
Da anni

**24. What does the pain feel like?**
Com´é il dolore?

**25. Acute**
Punge

**26. Dull**
Cupo

**27. Dragging**
Tira

**28. Did the pain develop slowly?**
   Il dolore si è sviluppato piano

**29. Did the pain develop fast?**
   Il dolore si è sviluppato subito?

**30. Does the pain last for a long time?**
   Il dolore tiene a lungo?

**31. Several seconds**
   Dei secondi

**32. Several minutes**
   Dei minuti

**33. Several hours**
   Delle ore

**34. Several days**
   Dei giorni

**35. Did you have an accident?**
  Ha avuto un incidente?

**36. Have you had treatment yet?**
  È stato visitato già?

**37. Yes**
  Si

**38. No**
  No

**39. Do you have high blood pressure?**
  Lei soffre di ipertensione

**40. Do you have diabetes?**
  Ha il diabete?

**41. Are you dizzy?**
  Soffre di vertigini?

**42. Are you pregnant?**

Lei è incinta?


**43. What month?**

Di quanti mesi?


**44. Do you take pain killers?**

Prende dei antidolorifici?


**45. Do you take blood thinning medication?**

Lei si prende dei medicamenti per diluire il sangue?


**46. Do you have problems with your thyroid?**

Ha dei problemi con la tiroide?


**47. Do you have heart problems?**

Ha dei problemi con il cuore?


**48. Do you have a headache?**

Ha dei dolori di testa?

**49. Did you have surgery?**
È stato operato?

**50. When did you have surgery?**
Quando é stata l′operazione?

**51. A few days ago**
Da giorni

**52. A few months ago**
Da mesi

**53. A few years ago**
Da anni

**54. You have to see a doctor.**
Lei ha bisogno di andare dal dottore

**55. Does it hurt when you are moving?**
Ha dei dolori nel momento di sforzo?

**56. Do you have pain while resting?**
   Ha dei dolori nel momento di riposo?

**57. When does it hurt most? When is the pain worst?**
   In quale situazioni sono piú forte i dolori?

**58. In the morning**
   La mattina

**59. In the evening**
   La sera

**60. At night**
   La notte

**61. Always the same**
   Sempre uguale

**62. While going up**
   Quando sale

**63. While going down**

Quando scende

**64. Going up the stairs**

Quando sale le scale

**65. Going down the stairs**

Quando scende le scale

**66. While sitting for a long time**

Mentre è seduta alungo?

**67. After sitting for a long time**

Dopo che è stato seduto molto tempo?

**68. While doing small movements?**

Mentre dei muovimenti piccoli?

**69. Were you in the hospital / in rehab?**

E stato all´ ospedale, in casa di cura?

**70. For how long?**
Per quando tempo?

**71. Several days**
Alcuni giorni

**72. Several weeks**
Alcune settimane

**73. Several months**
Alcuni mesi

**74. When did you get discharged from the hospital?**
Quando è stato dimesso dall´ospedale?

**75. Yesterday**
Ieri

**76. The day before yesterday**
Avanti ieri

**77. A few days ago**
   Un paio di giorni fa

**78. How many?**
   Quanti?

**79. A few weeks ago**
   Alcune settimane fa

**80. A few months ago**
   Alcuni mesi fa

# Massage

Massaggio

**1. Please get undressed**
Si spogli per favore

**2. Can you please take off your top?**
Puo togliersi il disopra?

**3. Can you please take off your pants?**
Puo togliersi il pantalone?

**4. Can you please take off your skirt?**
Puo togliersi la gonna?

**5. Lie down on your back**
Si puo sdraiarsi sulla schiena

**6. Lie down on your stomach**
Si puo sdraiarsi sulla pancia

**7. Lie down on your right side**
   Si puo sdraiarsi sul´lato destro

**8. Lie down on your left side**
   Si puo sdraiarsi sul´lato sinistro

**9. This is for your head**
   La testa qui per favore

**10. Would you like a blanket?**
   Vuole una coperta?

**11. Are you cold?**
   Ha freddo?

**12. Are you too warm?**
   Ha caldo?

**13. Put your right arm down**
   Appoggi il braccio destro, sotto

**14. Put your right arm next to your head**
Appoggi il braccio destro, sopra

**15. Align your right arm alongside your body**
Appoggi il braccio destro verso il corpo

**16. Put your left arm down**
Appoggi il braccio sinistro, sotto

**17. Put your left arm next to your head**
Appoggi il braccio sinistro, sopra

**18. Align your left arm alongside your body**
Appoggi il braccio sinistro verso il corpo

**19. Sit down please.**
Si sieda per favore

**20. Relax your shoulders**
Lasci sciolte la spalla

**21. Please look straigt ahead**
Guardi avanti

**22. Does it hurt?**
Le fà male?

**23. Do I hurt you?**
Le faccio male?

**24. Show me where it hurts.**
Mi faccia vedere dove le fà male

**25. Is the pressure ok?**
Va bene la pressione cosi?

**26. Yes?**
SI?

**27. No?**
NO?

## 28. Harder?
Piu forte?

## 29. Softer?
Piu piano?

## 30. Better?
Meglio?

## 31. Worse?
Peggio?

# Manual therapy

## Terapia manuale

**1. Please get undressed**
   Si spogli per favore

**2. Can you please take off your top?**
   Puo togliersi il disopra?

**3. Can you please take off your pants?**
   Puo togliersi il pantalone?

**4. Can you please take off your skirt?**
   Puo togliersi la gonna?

**5. Where does it hurt?**
   Dove ha dei dolori?

**6. Has it improved since the last treatment?**
   Va meglio dal´ultima terapia?

**7. Has it gotten worse?**

È peggiorato?

**8. Has the pain increased?**

Ha più dolori di prima?

**9. Has the pain gotten less?**

Ha meno dolori di prima?

**10. Where does it hurt now?**

Dove ha adesso il dolore?

**11. Stand on one leg please.**

Resti su una gamba

**12. Please stand on the other leg now.**

Adesso su l'altra gamba

**13. Stand on your heels**

Si metta sui calcagni

**14. Stand on your tiptoes**

Resti sulle punte dei piedi

**15. Sit down please**
Si sieda

**16. Round your back**
Si metta awolto su se stesso

**17. Put your chin to your chest**
Avvolga la testa

**18. Does it pull?**
Le tira?

**19. Is it painful?**
Fà male?

**20. Is the pain less now?**
Così di meno?

**21. Is the pain worse now?**
Così di più?

**22. Better?**
Meglio?

**23. Worse?**
   Peggio?

**24. Put your head back**
   Alzi la testa

**25. Lift your head up, look up**
   Alzi la testa in sù / guardi in sù

**26. Put your head down, look down**
   In giù la testa / Guardi in giù

**27. Turn your head to the left**
   Giri la testa a sinistra

**28. Turn your head to the right**
   Giri la testa a destra

**29. Tilt your head to the left**
   Pieghi la testa a sinistra

**30. Tilt your head to the right**
   Pieghi la testa a destra

**31. Relax**

Rilassare

**32. Do not help. I will do the movements, you relax**

Non aiuti, io faccio i movimenti, si rilassi

**33. Put your arms up**

In alto le braccia

**34. Put your right arm up**

In alto il braccio destro

**35. Put your right arm down**

Abbassi il braccio destro

**36. Put your left arm up**

In alto il braccio sinistro

**37. Put your left arm down**

Abbassi il braccio sinistro

**38. Bend your leg**

Piegare la gamba

**39. Extend your leg**
   Stendere la gamba

**40. Bend your knee**
   Piegare il ginocchio

**41. Extend your knee**
   Stendere il ginocchio

**42. Lift your leg**
   Alzare la gamba

**43. Lie on your back**
   Si può sdraiarsi sulla schiena

**44. Lie on your stomach**
   Si può sdraiarsi sulla pancia

**45. Lie on your right side**
   Si può sdraiarsi sul´lato destro

**46. Lie on your left side**
   Si può sdraiarsi sul´lato sinistro

**47. Put your head here, please**
La testa qui per favore

**48. Sit down**
Si sieda

**49. Please participate with ease**
Faccia anche lei i movimienti insieme

**50. Press against my resistance**
Spinga verso la mia resistenza

**51. Press harder**
Spinga più forte

**52. Press not so hard**
Spinga più piano

**53. This is an exercise to do at home**
Questo è un esercizio per farlo a casa

**54. Bend your legs and pull your knees to your thighs**
Le gambe erette

**55. Tighten your Abdomen**
Tendere la pancia

**56. Squeeze your buttocks**
Tendere il sedere

**57. Tense your legs**
Tendere le gambe

**58. Tense your arms**
Tendere le braccia

**59. Relax**
Rilasciare

**60. It might hurt a little**
Puo essere che fà male un pó

**61. I will show you first, then you repeat**
Io le faccio vedere, lei lo rifá

**62. Do 3 sets with 10 repetitions**
Lo fá 3 volte 10

**63. Do 3 sets with 15 repetitions**
Lo fá 3 volte 15

**64. Do 3 sets with 20 repetitions**
Lo fá 3 volte 20

**65. Do 3 sets with 30 repetitions**
Lo fá 3 volte 30

**66. Once a week**
Una volta la settimana

**67. Twice a week**
Due volte la settimana

**68. Three times a week**
Tre volte la settimana

**69. Once a day**
Una volta al giorno

**70. Twice a day**
Due volte al giorno

**71. Three times a day**

Tre volte al giorno


**72. Do the exercise in front of a mirror**

Faccia questi esercizi d´avanti lo specchio


**73. Sit down in front of a mirror**

Si sieda d´avanti lo specchio


**74. Stand in front of a mirror**

Si metti in piedi d´avanti lo specchio


**75. It is not supposed to hurt**

Questo non deve far del male


**76. This is not supposed to happen**

Questo non deve succedere

# PNF

## Rieducazione propriocettiva

**1. Lie on your back**
   Si può sdraiarsi sulla schiena

**2. Lie on your stomach**
   Si può sdraiarsi sulla pancia

**3. Lie on your right side**
   Si può sdraiarsi sul lato destro

**4. Lie on your left side**
   Si può sdraiarsi sul lato sinistro

**5. Put your head here, please**
   La testa qui per favore

**6. I will show you what the movement should look like**
   Le faccio vedere il movimento come deve fare

**7. I will do the movement, relax your arm**
   Io faccio il movimento e lei lascia il braccio rilasciato

**8. I will do the movement, relax your leg**
   Io faccio il movimento e lei lascia la gamba rilasciata

**9. Press against my resistance now**
   Spinga verso la mia resistenza

**10. Open your hand and extend your fingers**
   Apri le dita, la mano

**11. Close your hand aroung mine**
   Chiuda le dita, la mano

**12. Extend your arm**
   Stendere il gomito

**13. Bend your elbow**
   Piegare il gomito

**14. Put your leg up**
   La gamba sù

**15. Put your leg down**
   La gamba giù

**16. Tense your leg in this direction**
   Tendere la gamba in questa direzione

**17. Bend your knee**
   Piegare il ginocchio

**18. Extend your knee**
   Stendere il ginocchio

**19. Bend your hips**
   Piegare i fianchi

**20. Extend your hips**
   Stendere i fianchi

**21. Relax**
Rilassare

**22. More**
Di piú

**23. Less**
Di meno

**24. Harder**
Piú forte

**25. Softer**
Piú debole

**26. Slower**
Piú piano

**27. Faster**
Piú svelto

**28. Press upward**
   Spingere in sù

**29. Press downward**
   Spingere giù

**30. Now in the other direction**
   Adesso nell´altra direzione

**31. Towards your opposite shoulder**
   Direzione di fronte la spalla

**32. Towards your opposite hip**
   Direzione di fronte ai fianchi

**33. Towards the ear**
   Direzione verso l´orechio

**34. Towards the nose**
   Direzione verso il naso

**35. Towards the window**
Direzione verso la finestra

**36. Towards the door**
Direzione verso la porta

**37. Towards the wall**
Direzione verso il muro

**38. Towards the clock**
Direzione verso l'orologio

# **Mulligan**

## Mulligan

**1. Show me which movement causes the pain**
Mi faccia vedere quale movimento fa male

**2. Relax**
Si rilassi

**3. Repeat the movement once more**
Ripeta il movimento

**4. Is it better?**
Meglio così?

**5. Do you have pain going upstairs?**
Ha dei dolori quando sale le scale?

**6. Do you have pain going downstairs?**
Ha dei dolori quando scende le scale?

**7. Is it better like this?**

Meglio così?

**8. You are not supposed to be in pain. Please say Stop if it hurts**

Non deve avere dolore, se fà male mi dica "stop".

**9. If the strap hurts, I can put a pad between you and the strap**

Se le fà male la cinta, metto un cuscino in mezzo.

**10. You can do this exercise with a towel at home**

A casa puo fare questo esercizio con un asciuga mano

**11. you can do this exercise at home with an elastic band**

A casa può fare questo esercizio con una gomma terapotica

**12. You can do this exercise at home with a stick**

A casa può fare questo esercizio con un bastone

**13. The ball can be purchased at a sporting goods store**

Questa palla la può comprare in un negozio sportivo

**14. The elastic band can be purchased at a sporting goods store**

Questa gomma terapotica la puó comprare in un negozio sportivo

**15. It should be red**

Deve essere rosso

**16. It should be green**

Deve essere verde

# Exercises

Esercizi

**1. Bend**
Piegare

**2. Extend**
Stendere

**3. Flex**
Tendere

**4. Relax**
Rilasciare

**5. Move your buttocks backwards**
Il sedere in dietro

**6. tense your abdomen / do not relax**
Tendere la pancia / lasciare teso

**7. Remain like this for a few seconds, then relax**

Rimanga così un paio di secondi, poi si rilasci

**8. Do not move**

Non ci deve essere un movimento

**9. This is for your coordination**

Questo e per la coordinazione

**10. Do 3 sets with 10 repetitions**

Lo fá 3 volte 10

**11. Do 3 sets with 15 repetitions**

Lo fá 3 volte 15

**12. Do 3 sets with 20 repetitions**

Lo fá 3 volte 20

**13. Do 3 sets with 30 repetitions**

Lo fá 3 volte 30

**14. Take a break between the sets**

Faccia delle pause durante le sedute

**15. A few seconds**

Un paio di secondi

**16. A few minutes**

Un paio di minuti

**17. How many**

Quanto?

**18. Once a week**

Una volta la settimana

**19. Twice a week**

Due volte la settimana

**20. Three times a week**

Tre volte la settimana

**21. Once a day**

Una volta al giorno

**22. Twice a day**

Due volte al giorno

**23. Three times a day**

Tre volte al giorno

**24. Do the exercise while standing in front of a mirror**

Faccia questo esercizio davanti lo specchio

**25. Sit in front of the mirror**

Si sieda davanti lo specchio

**26. Stand in front of the mirror**

In piedi davanti lo specchio

**27. This is for strengthening**

Questo é per rinforzare

**28. Do it at home every day**

Farlo ogni giorno a casa

**29. Do the exercises in front of the mirror so that you can correct yourself**

Faccia questi esercizi davanti lo specchio, per correggere se stesso

**30. This is not supposed to happen**
   Questo non deve succedere

**31. This is wrong**
   Questo é sbagliato

**32. This is correct**
   Cosi é giusto

**33. Slow**
   Piano

**34. Slower**
   Più piano

**35. Fast**
   Veloce

**36. Faster**
   Più veloce

**37. don't jerk**
   Non a strappi

**38. Your are not supposed to be in pain during the exercise**

Non deve avere dei dolori mentre fa l'esercizio

**39. If you are in pain doing the exercise please stop and tell me next time you are here.**

Se ha dei dolori mentre fa l'esercizio, lasci stare e melo dica la prossima volta

**40. Did you do the exercises?**

Ha fatto gli esercizi?

**41. Did you feel any pain?**

Ha avuto dei dolori mentre ha fatto l'esercizio?

**42. Show me where it hurt?**

Mi faccia vedere dov' era il dolore?

**43. Show me how you do the exercises?**

Mi faccia vedere come ha fatto l'esercizio.

**44. Stand on your right leg**

Stia in piedi sulla gamba destra

**45. Stand on your left leg**
   Stia in piedi sulla gamba sinistra

**46. Stand on one leg**
   Stia in piedi su una gamba

**47. This is for balance**
   Questo é per l´equilibrio

**48. Try not to move**
   Provi a non traballare

**49. Try to include this exercise in your daily routine**
   Questo movimento puó farlo ogni giorno

# Gait Training

## Rieducazione mobile

**1. Stand straight**

Si metta diritto in piedi

**2. Take smaller steps**

Faccia dei passi più piccoli

**3. Take bigger steps**

Faccia dei passi più grande

**4. Take regular steps**

Faccia dei passi regolari

**5. Roll your foot from heel to toe**

Faccia scorrere il piede

**6. First on your heel, roll your foot, then press your foot forward to your toes**

Prima sul calcagno, poi scorra il piede, spinga il piede avanti con il davanti del piede

**7. The crutch goes on the same side as your injured leg**

Questo aiuto deve andare con la gamba malata

**8. Swing your arms loosely by your body**

Lasci andare le braccia penzolanti per il corpo

# Lymphatic drainage

## Linfodrenaggio

1. **The blood pressure cannot be taken on this arm nor can blood be drawn**

    Su questo braccio non si deve misurare la pressione né fare puntura

2. **Preferably you should not get hurt**

    Cerci di non ferirsi

3. **You are not allowed to take a hot bath or lie in the sun for too long**

    Non deve fare bagno caldo né stare molto al sole

4. **If you have a painful rash, see a doctor immediately**

    Se ha un sfogo doloroso, subito del medico

5. **Put your legs up multiple times per day**

    Metta piú tempo possibile al giorno le gambe alzate

**6. Put your leg up several times a day**
Metta piú tempo possibile al giorno la gamba alzata

**7. Put your arm up multiple times a day**
Metta piú tempo possibile al giorno il braccio alzato

**8. Do you have a surgical stocking?**
Ha una calza antitrombose?

**9. Do you have surgical stockings?**
Ha delle calze antitrombose?

**10. You have to wear the stocking every day**
La calza la deve portare ogni giorno

**11. You have to wear the stockings every day**
Le calze le deve portare ogni giorno

**12. You have to wear the stocking night and day**
La calza la deve portare giorno e notte

**13. You have to wear the stockings night and day**
Le calze le deve portare giorno e notte

**14. You shouldn't wear tight-fitting clothes**

Non deve portare dei vestiti stretti


**15. Lie on your back**

Si può sdraiarsi sulla schiena


**16. Lie on your stomach**

Si gira sulla pancia


**17. Can you lie on your stomach or would your rather sit?**

Si puó sdraiare sulla pancia o meglio sedersi?


**18. Sit?**

Sedersi?


**19. Put one leg up**

Alzi la gamba


**20. Put both legs up**

Alzi le gambe


**21. Slide a little towards me**

Scivoli un pó verso di me

**22. Slide to the left**

Scivoli verso sinistra

**23. Slide to the right**

Scivoli verso destra

**24. Slide up**

Scivoli verso la testa

**25. Slide down**

Scivoli verso i piedi

**26. Does it hurt?**

Fà male?

**27. It shouldn't hurt**

Non deve far male

# Electrotherapy

## Elettroterapia

**1. I will attach 2 electrodes**
   Le metto 2 elettrodi

**2. I will attach 4 electrodes**
   Le metto 4 elettrodi

**3. There is no electricity yet**
   Non scorre ancora corrente

**4. I will increase the electricity slowly**
   Giro piano ad alzere la corrente

**5. Tell me, as soon as you feel the electricity**
   Mi dica quando comincia a sentire la corrente

**6. Do you feel the electricity?**
   Sente la corrente?

**7. It should be comfortable**

Deve essere gradevole

**8. Is it comfortable?**

É gradevole?

**9. You should feel the electricity only slightly**

Deve sentire la corrente leggermente

**10. I will turn down the electricity until you can't feel it anymore**

Ora le giro la corrente giú finché non la sente piú

**11. It will take about 10 minutes**

Dura ca. 10 minuti

**12. It will take about 15 minutes**

Dura ca 15 minuti

**13. It will take about 20 minutes**

Dura ca. 20 minuti

**14. I will take off the electrodes once it is finished**
Quando é finito vengo é gli levo gli elettrodi

**15. If you have a problem, call me**
Se ha dei problemi, mi chiami

**16. I will be next-door**
Sono quí vicino

# Pelvic floor exercises

Esercizi per la Diaframma pelvico

### Short

1. **The pelvic floor is the muscle between your pubic bone and your tailbone**

   Il diaframma pelvico é il muscolo frá l'osso pubico e il coccige.

2. **Its function is mainly to close the openings there**

   La sua funzione é quella di chiudere le aperture che ci si trovano

3. **It works together with you abdominal muscles and your diaphragm**

   Lavora con i muscoli addominali e con il diaframma insieme.

4. **In order to strengthen your pelvic floor you have to use these muscles as well**

   Per questo bisogna far lavorare questi muscoli per rafforzare il diaframma pelvico.

5. **Try to tense your pelvic floor, acting like have to use the bathroom but you can't go**

   Provi a tendere il diaframma pelvico come se dovesse andare in bagno ma non puó.

## **Long**

1. **The pelvic floor is the muscle between ischial tuberosities, pubic and tailbone**

   Il diaframma pelvico é il muscolo che si trove trá l'osso ischio destro e sinistro, il coccige e l´osso pubico.

2. **The pelvic floor helps to control the function of urinating and bowel movement. With regular training you can prevent incontinence or lessen exiting problems**

   Il diaframma pelvico ha il compito di controllare la vostra fuori uscita di urina e feci. Per questo bisogna allenarlo regolarmente.

**3. In addition, the pelvic floor holds and supports the organs in your abdomen. That's why regular pelvic floor training works against prolapse problems**

Il diaframma pelvico dá supporto agli organi addominali da sotto, per questo con allenamento anticipa un abbassamento degli organi.

**4. To fulfill these functions, the pelvic floor works with the abdominal muscles and the diaphragm, which is the most important respiratory muscle.**

Per far sì che questi esercizi riecano il diaframma pelvico lavora con i muscoli addominali e il diaframma, il principale muscolo respiratorio.

**5. In order to strengthen your pelvic floor you have to use these muscles as well**

Per questo bisogna far lavorare i muscoli per far sí che il diaframma pelvico si rafforzi

**6. Try to tighten your pelvic floor, imagining closing your vagina and anus**

Provi a tendere il diaframma pelvico come se volesse chiudere l'ano e la sua vagina.

**7. Try to tighten your pelvic floor, acting like have to use the toilet but you can't go**

Provi a tendere il diaframma pelvico come se devesse andare in bagno me non puó.

**8. Inhale deeply. Exhale slowly tensing your abdominal muscles**

Aspiri profondamente e poi respiri piano tendere la pancia

**9. I will show you, and then you do it**

Le faccio vedere dopo lei lo rifá.

# Breathing therapy

## Riabilitazione respiratoria

**1. Inhale through your nose**
   Aspiri con il naso

**2. Exhale through your mouth**
   Respiri con la bocca

**3. I will show you, and then you do it**
   Le faccio vedere come deve fare, e lei lo rifá

**4. Slowly**
   Piano

**5. Slower**
   Più piano

**6. Fast**
   Veloce

**7. Faster**

Piú veloce

**8. Deeply**

Profondamente

**9. Deeper**

Più profondamente

**10. Casual**

Superficialmente

**11. More casually**

Più superficialmente

**12. Inhale more into your abdomen**

Respiri piu nella pancia

**13. Your abdomen should expand when inhaling**

La pancia deve gonfiarsi quando lei aspire

**14. Put your hands on your abdomen**

Mette le mani sulla pancia

**15. Put your hands on your ribcage**

Mette le braccia sul petto

**16. Your hands should be moving on your abdomen when inhaling**

Le sue mani si dovrebbero muovere dalli pancia quando lei aspire.

# Useful

Utile

**1. Hello**
Buon giorno

**2. Goodbye**
Ciao

**3. Please**
Prego

**4. Thank you**
Grazie

**5. Relax**
Rilasci

**6. Does it hurt?**
Fà male?

**7. Is it better now?**
   Meglio cosi?

**8. Harder?**
   Più forte?

**9. Yes**
   Si

**10. No**
   No

**11. I'm sorry, I can't understand you**
   Mi dispiace, ma non la capisco

# Thanks

I would like to thank all those who helped me to create the Little Physio book and application.

Thanks to the translators and the proof-readers, thanks to my family and my friends who have all participated in this adventure.

Thanks to those who helped with their voice on the apps and the videos.

Special thanks to my husband who programmed the apps for android and apple and for everything else too... :)

Thank you, dear reader for having bought this book or any of my other books.


If you have enjoyed Little Physio,
please leave comments on Amazon.

I would appreciate it very much :)

# Bibliography

- **Little Physio** from English into Spanish
- **Little Physio** from English into Italian
- **Little Physio** from English into French
- **Little Physio** from English into German
- **Little Physio** from English into Turkish

and

- **Big Little Physio** from English into Spanish, Italian, French, German and Turkish

www.ingramcontent.com/pod-product-compliance
Lightning Source LLC
Chambersburg PA
CBHW071802170526
45167CB00003B/1135